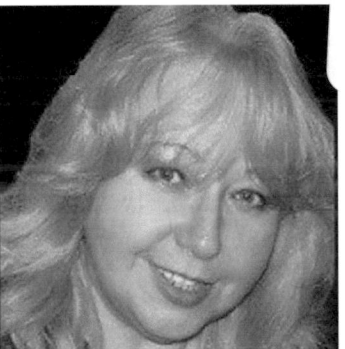

Jutta Schütz (Writer, journalist, psychologist, teacher) writes books that inspire, motivate and provide special insider knowledge. For more information on the author and her books see the publishers: A.S. Rosengarten-Verlag, tredition Hamburg, BoD Norderstedt.

http://www.jutta-schuetz-autorin.de/
info.jschuetz@googlemail.com

Preface

Dear Readers,

you bought this book because you believe that miracles sometimes happen in life.

I would like to point out that I am not a doctor of medicine.

These are my personal experiences with the disease - and how I've managed to get my blood sugar levels back into the normal range.

Every man or woman older than eighteen who is not incapacitated is responsible for him- or herself.

To date I don't need no pills or insulin.

Unfortunately, scientists are still arguing whether diabetes type two is curable or not.

Anyway, I am considered a maverick in relation to the diabetes type two, a rebel concerning Low Carb in the press.

The book comprises three parts:

- ❖ Diary
- ❖ Information
- ❖ Low-Carb Recipes

Jutta Schütz

DIABETES
Help yourself

3rd revised edition 2014

© 2014 author: Jutta Schütz
http://www.jutta-schuetz-autorin.de/
info.jschuetz@googlemail.com

© 2014 Publisher: BoD – Books on Demand, Norderstedt
Printed in Germany
3rd revised edition

ISBN: 978-3735757302

Bibliographic Information of the German National Library. The German National Library lists this publication in the German National Bibliography; detailed bibliographic data are available on the Internet at http://dnb.d-nb.de.

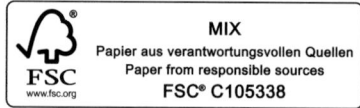

MIX
Papier aus verantwortungsvollen Quellen
Paper from responsible sources
FSC
www.fsc.org
FSC® C105338

Diary

➤ 31st July 2007

Today was a very terrible day for me. After a routine examination I received the diagnosis of diabetes type two from my family doctor! I had to pull myself together to be able to follow the doctor's instructions in total. He asked me whether I was often thirsty, but I said no. Similarly, I had no urge to constantly go to the toilet.

BUT: I had felt exhausted and tired for months and I could not even really explain my ever-changing depression. Three weeks later I should come back and he would set me on pills then, he told me in parting. I asked him what else I could do, and he answered I should leave the carbs off. During the twenty minute walk home I was in a fog, and I was very shocked.

I will now be diabetic? Why me?

I imagined the people who had to inject themselves with insulin daily, who I had always commiserated. And now I should also be among these people? Still shocked, I started my PC at home and informed me what diabetes is and how it is generated. When my husband came home from work, I had already read about it for hours. I knew that in the beginning of diabetes the symptoms may be absent entirely, and that the diabetes would develop gradually. One year ago, my blood counts were still in order.

At that time, another doctor told me that I would probably never fall ill on diabetes, because I had very good blood values. I remember the proverb: Never say never! I was so upset that I could not go to bed and sat down again and again in front of the PC and studied more Google-results.

The Diabetes Federation says: 1985, worldwide - 30 million people with diabetes. 10 years later there were already 150 million. Today (2009), there are already over 285 million.

➤ 01st August 2007

I had not slept well that night and I felt very, very bad. Immediately after my so-called breakfast - I ate nothing at all - I went back to the PC to read more. You don't have to know everything, but you should know where you can look to increase your knowledge. What did my doctor say? I should leave off the carbs! What are carbohydrates? In a report I read that carbs simply spoken are – sugar!

Certainly just like many other people I had known for a long time that sugar can be harmful for diabetics. Sugar is glucose and actually the most important carbohydrate in the body that provides the energy.

We eat sugar, it is converted into glucose, which is stored and consumed. In the report, they stressed that there are indigestible and digestible carbohydrates. The indigestibles would belong to the fiber and the digestibles split up in the intestine, are absorbed and then pass through the blood vessels to the cells. Important for the body is the constant supply of glucose. This glucose concentration is regulated by the hormone insulin. You find carbohydrates in plant products such as noodles, rice, bread (all cereals), vegetables and fruit. I spent the whole day to read medical reports on diet and still did not really know what I could eat. There were carbohydrates everywhere, with the exception of meat. It was even stated that one could get cancer by too many carbohydrates. I remembered now that in my childhood I always prayed before lunch:

"Pray the Lord's Prayer, our daily bread give us today ... ..", and my mother cut a cross with a knife into the back of the bread before she broached. In meat there are no carbohydrates, but I had heard for many years that it is not good to eat much meat. And what else should I eat now?

➢ 02nd August 2007

Today is my 47th Birthday! And I'm diabetic!

My God, what a drama, I thought. And I thought the same about my dear friend Inge, who had had this disease for ten years then and coped with it that well. That encouraged me a bit! I didn't want to celebrate that birthday. I canceled the party and informed all my friends. I could not eat cake anyway! Instead, I turned on the PC. Somehow I came upon a report, where it was maintained that the cholesterol level increases if a person eats too many carbohydrates. But hadn't it always been claimed that the cholesterol level increased by too many eggs and animal products?

The more I read, the more confused I became. I was totally scatter-brained because there were reports that you should eat a lot of wholemeal (and carbohydrates) and less animal fat and meat. These reports contradicted the opinions which alleged that the carbohydrates in the grain (bread, pasta), potatoes and rice are not good. How can someone who has not studied medicine get the picture? And even these trained scientists, doctors, professors had different opinions! Now I was completely confused.

➢ 03rd August 2007

My God, am I glad to have my friend Renate. She knew that I was not well for months and when I told her the diagnosis yesterday she answered that I should get in the car and pay her a visit in the Saarland with my family.

Step by step I did things like packing suitcases, housekeeping or cooking like in a fog. I was out of my mind, confused. When we arrived Saarlouis after two hours of driving, my friend kissed and hugged me a long time. To relax a bit, we two women went on a trip in Renate's big open-top car through the beautiful Saarland. It was good to feel the sun on my skin, the wind in my hair and to know my friend by my side.

➢ 06th August 2007

I was so happy that we had been in the web since Christmas. Without the Internet I wouldn't have learned that much. Who would buy a thousand non-fiction books? Apart from the money that they would cost.

I found a report about the fact that adults have too little lactase (an enzyme) to digest the milk sugar, lactose. Thus, the lactose is digested in the large intestine and leads to acidosis. I also read that some nutritionists warn of whole foods. But that is the opposite of what I had heard and read in former times! So, what was the right answer for me? I was even more confused. But in fact, I had already tried out the idea of eating less animal products, I had followed it for many years. At that time I thought it was healthy! I now had diabetes, perhaps because I ate too many carbohydrates? A report was submitted that cereal fiber (bran harm) the intestine, fiber from fruit and vegetables would be better, however.

According to Dr. Wolfgang Lutz you should consume only about six units of bread each day. That's about the daily sugar consumption of the brain. This means for every kg of body weight 0.8 g carbohydrate per day. That would be about 50-70 g carbs a day for a 70 kg man.

➢ 07th August 2007

This day I spent with my PC as well and I didn't care about the undone housework. My God, what should I do? Some nutritionists advise this way, others the opposite. And all of them were studied with the same degree. If they didn't agree with each other, what could I say and do? I just had to give it a try because after all, I am a self-responsible person.

➢ 08th August 2007

After the return from the Saarland I eat for breakfast two eggs, a tomato and a raw carrot every day. Lunch is no problem, I simply leave off the side dishes such as pasta, rice and potatoes. In the evening I eat salad and sausages or meat. But I miss the bread at breakfast and I'm wondering how I should hold on.

➢ 09th August 2007

It is becoming increasingly difficult to live without bread. Should I perhaps eat such a wholemeal roll? Whole grain is still healthy! Just now I have read about it in a magazine. BUT: I have not forgotten all the reports that told me the opposite. No, I don't want to eat wholemeal. This morning I ate a natural yogurt and an additional apple. Somehow I feel that I am suffering from withdrawal symptoms because I feel a little overexcited as if I was charged with electric current and now don't know where to put all this energy. I have read that if you reduce the carbohydrates, the body assimilates more protein. Of course, I now eat more animal products, I somehow have to replace the grain. Oh dear, I get scared that it will hurt me. But I have no feeling of fullness longer after the meals and this constant flatulence has improved. I am surprised that I suddenly wake up around five in the morning without an alarm clock and get up much better. I still spend hours on the PC to read about nutrition, the human body, the organs and metabolism. Mankind is genetically much better adapted to animal fats than to vegetable oils. It is stressed that low-fat diets make you sick.

➢ 10th August 2007

For several days I haven't eaten bread. I miss the rolls every morning and it is difficult for me to stand that. For hours, I'm doing more research with the PC again and this time a report confuses me that tells, fruit are not as healthy as it is always said. Revitalize an African fruit in a hot climate, however, but they would devitalise an Eskimo. Fruit would not be good for every man. The hotter the climate, the better compliant is a fruit. It is recommended to eat the fruit sober in any case.

➢ 11th August 2007

I feel like doing sports again because I don't have to gasp any more if I go up the stairs. I also notice that my pants are made on. I should really go and stand on the scales. A fright!

I lost four kilos. I am not sick, am I? How can I lose weight although I ate a large portion of chicken salad in the evening? In the past I had often forborn having a dinner and only eaten one slice of bread. And what I also noticed, I haven't had to take any tablets against heartburn for a few days. These acid blockers had been my constant companion in recent years. They had always told me that I get heartburn from animal products. I am now very confused.

A report claims that bread is to blame that so many people have gastrointestinal problems. That is because of the phosphorus, due to the gluten, but also because of the heated starch. This strength would ferment and therefore constitute an excellent food for fungi and bacteria.

➢ 12th August 2007

I miss the rolls in the morning more and more and I'm almost fed up with the curd cheese and the eggs. I really don't like breakfast anymore and cook an early lunch instead. But that is no solution. BUT: I feel better now from day to day since I've been leaving out these carbohydrates.

The PC is now my daily companion and I read and read. Today I found an article that it is best to eat raw meat! The juice that comes from a roast (even meat soup), would be harmful. The spill should be poured away. And what happens to the beef soup I like so much? Well, if I still eat it two times a year, it cannot hurt. But raw meat? No thanks. This can't convince me anyway. Finally, my attention was attracted by a sentence at the end of a report saying: Who really wants, finds a way, who does not want finds an excuse.

➢ 13th August 2007

I'm still up at 5 o´clock in the morning, without the need of an alarm clock and I'm wide awake at once. My husband, who always had to wake me before is surprised and cares about me. But I feel alright all day and even think about jogging again. My God, I used to jog twice a week for up to 15 km in former times.

At the moment I leave out breakfast because I cannot see any eggs, yogurt, cottage cheese and sausage any more. I'm beginning to worry about my cholesterol because I eat a lot more animal products. But I also eat a lot more raw carrots, peppers, cucumbers, lettuce, tomatoes and vegetables. I want to do without oil so far and now put the meat in the already hot frying pan. Especially poultry and meat can be fried very well without oil. In the evening, after my daughter is in bed, I regularly go to my PC to get further information. Here I came across a report that is written in a forum. A woman reported that she was informed by her doctor half a year ago about the low-carb diet because her cholesterol grade was over 280. Within two months, it was down to 250 and her blood pressure and her previously elevated uric acid levels had normalized. What kind of a diet is this low-carb diet?

➢ 14th August 2007

This morning I went to my doctor due to a blood sample and they measured again my sober blood sugar levels. From 175 (at 31.07.07) it has declined to 150.

My doctor was amazed and asked me what I had done. He actually wanted to prepare me for tablets, but now he wanted to wait for the new result from the laboratory. He gave me a blood glucose meter and the nice receptionist taught me every detail. I shall now note a daily profile for several days. I am doing better and better. My depression is gone completely and I feel much better.

But I do still have Type Two Diabetes? I'm sick! Also, I notice again that I still do not need acid blockers. Since yesterday evening I've read in a forum (in fact it's a forum for weight loss), many reports by diabetics who have received better values by low-carb. Others write that they lost many pounds by this diet and feel better than ever before. I 'm keen on my results on the 24th will be.

➢ 15th August 2007

I have started to eat a yogurt and an apple for breakfast again. For lunch there is a cauliflower with cheese and an additional salad. In the evening, I would enjoy meat and eat two sausages and a salad. From now on, I decide from the gut. Of course, I read again in this forum about low-carbohydrate diets. There are the initials LC, that means low carb. They advise to have only three meals a day and to make sure that there is a break of five hours between them. This would avoid un-controlled grazing.

➢ 16th August 2007

Today is the first day I will only have three meals. Let's see how it works. When shopping this morning I came across a bakery and it smelled so delicious of fresh rolls. My God, I would have liked to bite into a piece of bread or like a juicy piece of pastry (in the Saarland we call them coffee bits). In the evening I read in this forum that if one wants to lose weight quickly, he should have an only maximum of 35 carbs per day. Who wants to keep his weight can eat 60 CH (carbohydrates allowed to eat).

➢ 17th August 2007

I find it very difficult to cope with the three meals, but I console myself with the fact that I can eat so much that I'm full up after every meal. Strangely, I am faster full up anyway since I've reduced the carbohydrates.

The cravings have disappeared completely, I have no more bloating and the slight dizziness of the beginning is gone too.

➢ 18th August 2007

I went shopping in the supermarket this morning. For the first time I read the carbohydrate information on the foods and not the calories table. There were pickles that have ten g carbohydrates on 100 g, while other cucumbers have only 2 g on100 g. Yogurt has eight g carbohydrates per 100 g, cottage cheese on the other hand has only half of that. In the forum I've read that one can also nibble nuts in between. I had always avoided them because of their calories. Now I stood in front of the shelf and looked for peanuts. And here you have to be careful too, since there are also those with shells or with glutamate. I also bought a can of macadamia nuts that have even less carb than peanuts. You can eat 50 g of nuts a day without a problem.

➢ 19th August 2007

For breakfast this morning I made American scrambled eggs and bacon. In addition I served a large plate of raw carrots, peppers, tomatoes, cucumbers, radishes, all cut into stripes. Later, we went on a long bike ride. We were full up until the early evening. In the evening I could rummage in the recipes from the forum and was dumbfounded that you can bake rolls with almond flour. But don't they taste sweet? I knew ground almonds only in a sweet pastry. I'm going to buy all the ingredients tomorrow.

➢ 20th August 2007

In the morning my blood sugar was at 120. I was happy. Thus, this diet called low-carb can't be that wrong! But what about my cholesterol level?

After my breakfast, with cottage cheese and apple pieces, I made my way to go shopping. Of course I was very curious to see how the rolls would taste.

Recipe

Ingredients:

3 eggs (stir until foamy), 120 g yogurt

1 tbsp cottage cheese, 50 g melted butter

1 teaspoon baking soda, ½ teaspoon salt

400 g ground almonds, 100 g sunflower seeds, 100 g sesame seeds

Procedure: But instead of filling in a cake pan I put the batter into the muffin form. At 160 degrees I baked them about 40-45 minutes. It smelled so wonderful! I was very curious what their taste would be like. They tasted super delicious. I could not wait to try them as a roll substitute. I added some butter, which I could eat again, and crowned the low-carb bread with cheese and a few slices of cu-cumber.

Simply super! My God, now I finally had bread for breakfast again. And the next time I'm simply going to bake a double quantity and freeze it.

➢ 21st August 2007

My breakfast this morning was just great. I am absolutely delighted. I cut the rolls in the middle and ate one half with salami and the other one with cheese. I added half a red pepper and a tomato. Was that delicious! Today, I got a high praise from my friend Claudia for my perseverance. Yes, it's even easier now since I've found something like a bread substitute. Even my family likes this low-carb bread.

➢ 22nd August 2007

My evening program now consists of looking around the forum for more recipes and reviews. And it's also getting clearer for me what such a low-carb diet is like. They say that you should drink decaffeinated coffee because the caffeine will hinder weight loss. And it is similar in all the various light-cola beverages.

➢ 23rd August 2007

This morning I was again able to speak my table prayer: Our Father, give us our daily bread ....These grain-rolls also taste great with cottage cheese and radish on them. I blossom new again and have continued to write my novel which I had parked in the drawer for two years.

➢ 24th August 2007

My blood sugar is around 118 in the morning. Isn't that super? My husband and my daughter are also happy about it and inspire me to continue. Maybe I don't need to take tablets?

➢ 25th August 2007

I'm getting more courageous in baking and so I bought chickpea flour in a health food shop. I want to make pizza because I miss it. Of course, my family will have to try it, too.

Recipe:

Ingredients:

4 egg (stir until foamy), 250 g chickpea flour

A pinch of salt, ¼ liter of mineral water (or more)

Procedure: I mixed the dough and diluted it with a little water and then let it rest for about half an hour. When they were baked, I appplied tomato paste from a tube on the thin pancakes and finished them with fresh tomatoes, herbs, thin slices of mushrooms, a few slices of salami and cheese on top. In 20 minutes they were baked at 200 degrees. My husband indeed meant that they tasted not like real pizza, but that they also were good. I think they are a great substitute for pizza.

➢ 26th August 2007

Today I'm going to bake a supply of the grain rolls and the chick-pea pancakes and freeze it. I had a blood sugar degree of 110 this morning, thus this low-carb food doesn't hurt me. In Google, there are plenty of reports about low-carb and also many books about it. I have really dear friends with whom I can talk about my main subject low-carb. They encourage me to go on with it and are surprised that there is such an enormous change in diet.

➢ 27th August 2007

I miss neither the "normal" bread any longer nor pizza. BUT: I would like to eat a piece of cake again. Unfortunately, baking a cheesecake went wrong yesterday. The recipe I had found in a forum sounded so delicious. The cake collapsed back upon itself after baking and tasted like rubber. No, you could not really eat it.

➢ 28th August 2007

Renate just called me and asked me if I was still doing this low-carb diet. She said she could not do without her beloved rice or potatoes and praised me that I was so adamant. At coffee time, I would really like a piece of cake! I'm going to try these cookies of which they were raving in this forum.

Recipe:

Ingredients:

6 eggs stirred very foamy, 180 g butter, melted

1 packet baking powder, 4 tablespoons liquid sweetener

1 packet Vanilla flavoring, 200 g ground almonds

200 g of protein powder

Procedure: Bake 30 minutes at 180 degrees.

But what is this protein powder and where can I get it? In the forum they told me you can get the powder in many major super-markets for about € 8-10 and that is considered a flavor substitute for low-carb baked goods. 100 g have about 1.5 CH!

➢ 29th August 2007

My world is almost back in order. I'm feeling great, like I hadn't for a long time. I could hug everyone and I am so glad that I found these nutritional changes. Today I am quite sure that was the best thing that happened to me recently. The diagnosis of diabetes has lost its horror for me. And these cookies are just mega super, super delicious! This afternoon I tested three cookies on a small coffee with a little milk.

➢ 30th August 2007

This morning I went to my GP again and he was more than satisfied with me. I had to tell him what diet I'm doing. He decided that for the time being I don't need to take any pills and I should register in the diabetic training.

➢ 31st August 2007

My friend Helga Schittek, the crime writer (Riemenschneider series) from Bad Neuenahr, told me today that an acquaintance got much better rheumatism values by such a "low-carbohydrate diet" and could reduce her tablets in half. Wow, I thought, even in this case low carb works well! In Google I found yet another posting that the positive low-carb effect has been reported by migraine patients as well.

➢ September 2007

I'm well supported by my family and my dear friends who praise me again and again and find it great that I can live like this. Almost all of them tell me that they could not even get along without bread, potatoes and Co. But, it works! I'm the best example. I don't look at the diagnosis "diabetes" in a negative way anymore, but it was probably the hammer from the top, that I had to change something!

➢ 03. September 2007

Today I first baked a cake.

Recipe:

Ingredients:

5 egg (stir until foamy), 100 g butter, melted

1 pack Vanilla flavoring, 2 tablespoons liquid sweetener

250 g ground almonds, 1 pack baking powder

3 heaped tablespoons good protein powder

3 heaped tablespoons mascarpone well

3 heaped tablespoons good cottage cheese

Procedure: Bake at 160 degrees about 40-50 minutes.

My God, that was the best cake I have ever eaten.

➢ 04th September 2007

Of course, I had a piece of cake for breakfast today and I added two tablespoons of cottage cheese. Very, very, yummy, I can tell. The side effect of this diet, which is not a diet but a change in diet, has brought me six kg less on the scale. That's a positive effect!

➤ 05th September 2007 - 22 September 2007

I live "without exception," according to the guidelines of the low-carb diet with approximately 40-50 CH per day. For breakfast there are alternately soft-boiled eggs or a grain bread, biscuits, or even a piece of cake, cream cheese, cottage cheese or yogurt with fruit.

➤ 23rd September 2007

Last night I came across reports that confused me again. Again I don't know for sure now if I'm on the right track with my low-carb diet. I feel so helpless and I'm torn. For lunch, I now have poultry in the oven and in addition there will be a raw food dish and a cauliflower without sauce, just with a little butter. For dinner, there is very little chicken salad with mayonnaise and iceberg lettuce.

➤ 24th September 2007

When I was informed about my blood degrees by my doctor today, I smiled from ear to ear. I think I hadn't had such good blood tests for a long time. Also, I had lost seven kg in weight - without going hungry anyway! Of course my doctor wanted to know exactly how I did it and I told him about the low-carb diet. When we parted, he praised me again and said that I was on the right track.

➤ 15th October 2007

My doctor doesn't want to lose sight of me. So I gave him some of my blood and he praised me again. All right! Even the daily profile I did at home was very good. He now enrolled me in the health program of my health insurance and I should join a diabetes training as well.

➤ 05th November 2007

I got it over the first day of diabetic training and I am very disappointed. The ladies did competently do the full monty, but unfortunately not in my diet. In the evening I then told my family and my friends that I'm the only one in this course who doesn't need pills or insulin.

➤ 06th November 2007

All participants were surprised that I had normal blood values because of a low-carb diet of which no one had heard yet. But unfortunately they did not let me tell too much. I was told that classes had to go on now. From then on, one lady looked always very seriously at me, when she told of carbohydrates the other participants could eat yet. She said that they could eat a small portion of potatoes, rice, pasta or bread. And every time she met an incredulous inner shake of the head from me.

➤ 07th November 2007

Most of all I would not go into this training anymore because I didn't learn useful facts for my diet. I often wanted to talk about my diet, but they didn't let me. I was also disappointed by the participants, because they weren't interested in how I do my diet. I could not believe that these people would rather swallow pills than change something in their diet.

➤ 08th November 2007

This morning, an older lady wasn't alright. Obviously, she had eaten a bit less carbohydrates, but not paid attention on her dose of medication. They measured a blood sugar of only 60. She was given glucose quickly and told that she should eat more in the future. She answered that she had frequently such deep measurements and they told her that she should eat more.

And I asked the counselor why they shouldn't change the medication! Only now I had mentioned that they recommended her to take only half a tablet a day. Then, the training director told me that the brain needed the carbohydrates anyway! After such a long time, I'm certainly gaga already! My arguments that I got my carbs even with vegetables, fruit, cottage cheese, or yogurt, they could not break, but would not elaborate on it.

➤ 09th November 2007

It is important that diabetics do sports! This was taught in this course, too, and I have to concede these leaders absolutely to this point. At the end of this course, I was the only one who held fast to the diet with low-carb. All others eat their though few carbohydrates in "small" portions of potatoes, rice, noodles, and continue to think that wholemeal bread is so healthy that it does not harm diabetic patients.

➢ 17th December 2007

Today I had another blood test and my doctor was happy. He told me that he would like to have more such patients like me. He said it was very, very difficult to persuade people to choose a different diet. Until now, I'm the only one concerning his patients who has done it with low-carb. To date, all diabetics I told about low carb were very surprised. On the other hand I am also very surprised that they have not inquired about alternatives.

➢ 19th December 2007

Someone asked me what I would do for Christmas when I couldn't bake cookies any more. Rubbish, I can bake fine cookies and even cakes. I'm well informed because of the Internet and I collected quite a lot of recipes and altered them after my fancy. Some recipes I could throw in the garbage and others I bake again and again.

Christmas is saved. These biscuits are so delicious that I had to pass the recipe many times.

➢ 29th February 2008

I'm doing very well. My blood sugar levels are better than ever before. I feel fit, do sports and I lost 18 kg to date. Of course, I'll regularly go for blood test and also do an occasional day profile. I wish all diabetic patients that they have the courage to try a few weeks with the low-carb diet. I'm sorry if this book looks like I'm touting for this diet.

It is my own experience that I was eager to tell you.

Additional informations

What are carbohydrates? A chemist would call them sugar or glucose.

In our body there are indigestible and digestible carbohydrates. Fiber are the indigestible carbohydrates. They go unchanged into the intestine. In the intestine, the digestible carbohydrates split up and go through the bloodstream to the cells. It is important to give the body a constant supply of glucose. The hormone insulin which is produced in the pancreas regulates the blood sugar.

Carbohydrates are found in: grain products (bread, pasta), fruits and vegetables, cheese, nuts and dairy products. Starch, for example, produced by heating (baking) of corn, potatoes, corn and rice gets inorganic, and hardened fats are harmful. This cereal fat (generated by the heat sets) releases transfats, which are very harmful. This then affects the hormonal balance and our glands. Many thyroid diseases are consequences of that.

The many carbohydrates cause hunger and you eat even more. The glucose-lowering hormone insulin is involved in the growth of these fat depots. If we eat too many carbohydrates, much insulin is produced, this can reduce the blood sugar level again and also inhibits fat burning in the muscles. The fat deposits in adipose tissue are promoted. Insulin is a masting hormone. If we eat too many CH, our body burns very little fat.

Some other terms concerning sugar: Glucose, Maltrodextrose, sucrose, fructose, raw sugar, brown sugar, fruit sugar, fructose, Farin, lactose, glucose syrup, dextrose, glucose, maltose, invert sugar, lactose.

Many people have an acidification of the tissue because of too many carbohydrates and not by eating too much meat and animal protein. Already in 1845, the British Nutrition researcher Haywood called bread and cereals "agents of death" and proved by many studies that bread and pasta lead to arteriosclerosis, blockages and calcifications. In 1996, the German Crohn's disease association published studies that showed that in a high fat diet the cholesterol and uric acid levels don't deteriorate. Dr. Russell of the Mayo Clinic in Rochester in 1920 successfully treated children suffering from epilepsy. Today, these ketogenic diet is used in over 45 countries, in Zurich even in a children's hospital. To this day there are no medication studies with similar results.

The liver produces ketone particles during ketosis and these may reduce the epileptic hyperactivity of the brain cells. Thomas Seyfried from Boston College found that in mice with brain tumors with ketogenic food, the tumors grew more slowly. Doctors and researchers discuss whether this diet could have positive effects also on Alzheimer's and Parkinson's. There are already studies with Alzheimer's or Parkinson's patients who showed positive effects with this diet.

19

If the body absorbs the carbohydrates too quickly, it could also lead to a migraine, which can occur when the vascular muscles are malnourished. Dr. Riegler explains: Only ten insulin-sugar particles can go through the cell door per minute, but 10.000 insulin-sugar particles want to pass through simultaneously. They trample each other. The consequence is that the cell receives nothing, and spasms.

The wheat lectin is suspected to promote diseases. The lectins are just a group of antibodies which clump red blood cells together and make our intestinal wall permeable. In whole grains the lectins remain because they are heat stable. Concerning white flour, these lectins with the embryo are largely separated. In addition, all forms of cereals also contain phytin and enzyme inhibitors that affect our digestion. If you heat (bake) this flour, minerals are dissolved and the body is heavily decalcified through this process. The result is osteoporosis. Fats and proteins are also altered by heating and in-completely decomposed in the stomach. The result is intestinal putrefaction and blast deposits.

Nutritionists hit choppy waters with the interpretation of the various study results and only recently the advocates of a low-carb diet increasingly gain more importance. There are already 100 different varieties of food pyramids and the scientists are still discussing which one is right.

Unfortunately, the layman can't recognize links between drug companies and the scientists, and the managers are clever. They are mostly educated nutrition or natural scientists. They spread studies in the media about healthy or not healthy diets for the benefit of their firms. The profit is huge!

All the civilizational diseases are a billion dollar business for the pharmaceutical industry, doctors and health insurers.

Sources (German books etc.)

DR KLAUS HOFFMANN - The disastrous grain acids, DR SOMOGYI - About the formation of calcium, phosphorus and vitamin D-deficiency, FRANZ KONZ - Also Langbein - The medical cartel, PETRA PLATE - Epilepsy - treatment by ketogenic diet, MR. ABEL HAYWOOD (1845) - Bread and cereals - substances of death, WILLIAM Banting (1797-1878) - Low-Carb Diet "Letter on corpulence", DR E. Densmore (1892), DR: Cordain LOREN (2004) - Cereals - the two-edged sword, DR DE LACY EVANS (1893) - The art to extend the life, PROF. DR WALTER C. WILLET, Professor of Medicine and Epidemiology, Harvard School of Public Health, Boston, ERIK RAUCH - The Carbohydrate case (Trias Verlag), WILLETT AND STAMPFER - Eat, Drink And Be Healthy, PHILADELPHIA Veterans Affairs Medical Center, Stern - et al. 2004, PROF. SUSANNE KLAUS (metabolic specialist), University of Potsdam, AUTHOR MAG: Walpurga WHITE, Austrian Society for Nutrition, William Banting - 1797 – 1878, PROF. DAVID LUDWIG, Harvard University, Dr WALTER Hartenbach - The Cholesterol-lie, the tale of bad cholesterol (Munich 2002), DR EHRENSPERGER - 2004 - writes about carbohydrates, Dr KLAUS HOFFMANN, DR WOLFGANG LUTZ - Life Without Bread, DCCV (GERMAN Crohn's Colitis, Lutz-diet study in 1996 under the direction of:, Prof. H. Lorenz-Meyer and, Prof. P. Bauer, OTTO HEINRICH WARBURG (Nobel laureate) Warburg effect - 1924 (tumor cells)

Low-Carb Recipes

Rolls with Cream Cheese

Ingredients:

- ➢ 8 eggs (stir until fluffy), 400 g cream cheese
- ➢ one bag of baking powder, 4 tablespoons ground flaxseed
- ➢ 2 tablespoons protein powder, 200 g ground almonds
- ➢ 2 cups sunflower seeds

Procedure: Separate eggs and beat the egg whites until stiff. Mix the egg yolk and all ingredients except for some sunflower seeds (for decoration) and fold in egg whites. Place 20 small heaps of dough with a tablespoon on a baking sheet lined with baking paper. Press the remaining sunflower seeds on the rolls. Bake at 175 degrees for 30-35 minutes until golden brown.

Breakfast Rolls

Ingredients:

- ➢ cool 250 g melted butter, 6 egg yolks
- ➢ 200 g of protein powder, 60 g linseed
- ➢ 700 g cream cheese, 1 sachet of baking powder

Procedure: Stir thoroughly and form about 16 pieces of bread. Bake 15-25 minutes at 175 degrees.

Crunchy breakfast rolls

Ingredients:

- ➢ 125 g melted butter, 4 egg yolks 35 g
- ➢ 200 g linseed Quark, 150 g protein powder (more or less)
- ➢ 1 sachet baking powder

Procedure: Stir everything together and form about 7-9 rolls and bake 15-20 minutes at 175 degrees.

Grain bread

Ingredients:

> ➤ 6 egg yolks, 200 g yogurt
>
> ➤ 100 g melted butter, 2 teaspoons baking soda
>
> ➤ 1 teaspoon salt, 800 g ground almonds
>
> ➤ 200 g sunflower seeds, 200 g sesame seeds

Procedure: Stir eggs and yogurt until creamy, add the remaining ingredients, stir again and fill, for example: in muffins (preferably with paper) and bake at 175 degrees about 40 minutes (in the cake pan about 1 hour).

Light bread (like dumplings)

Ingredients:

> ➤ Melt 250g of butter, let it cool
>
> ➤ 250 g quark, 6-7 eggs
>
> ➤ 200 g protein powder (or more), 1 sachet of baking powder, salt

Procedure: Mix everything together and form balls (about as big as a small apple), place them on a baking sheet (with parchment paper) and leave space between each ball! Bake at 200 degrees about 15-20 minutes.

Bread with bran

Ingredients:

> ➤ 6 eggs (separate four of them), 50 g melted butter
>
> ➤ 2 tablespoons sour cream or cottage cheese
>
> ➤ 60 g sunflower seeds, 30 g bran Spelt

- ➢ 60 g protein powder (or more), 2 tablespoons oil (Omega 3)
- ➢ 1 teaspoon baking soda, 1 teaspoon salt
- ➢ (By the soda, the sunflower seeds become green)

Procedure: Separate four eggs and stir the egg whites until stiff. Stir the egg yolks and the remaining whole eggs with the butter until fluffy. Then stir the remaining ingredients. Now add the soda. In the end, fold the beaten egg whites in. Put twelve heaps onto a baking sheet. Leave space between them. Bake at 175 degrees 25-30 minutes.

Pizza base

Ingredients:

- ➢ 4 egg yolks, 2 tablespoons hot water
- ➢ some salt, pepper and curry
- ➢ 200 grams ground almonds, 4 egg whites (or more)
- ➢ 1 sachet dried yeast, Oregano and a little tomato paste

Procedure: Stir egg yolks until fluffy and add the spices and the yeast. Mix the stirred egg whites with the almonds and fold into the egg yolk. Put the thinly rolled dough on a greased baking sheet. Then cover the dough with tomato paste and, for example, with mushrooms, salami or other ingredients. Finally the cheese. Bake at 200 degrees 20-30 minutes.

Yeast dough

Ingredients:

- ➢ 200 g ground almonds, 100 grams of protein powder (or more)
- ➢ 1 egg, 30 ml cream, 120 ml hot water
- ➢ 1 sachet of dried yeast, 15 g butter, melted
- ➢ 1 tablespoon oil, 2 tablespoons liquid sweetener or
- ➢ ½ teaspoon salt

Procedure: Stir water, cream and the egg and warm it. Then crumble the yeast into it. Sieve the ground almonds and the protein powder into a bowl, form into a

23

heap and put the yeast into a well. Leave the whole thing covered in a warm place for about 30 minutes. The butter, a little sweetener and a pinch of salt on the dough and knead the whole into a smooth dough. This dough will rise in a warm place until the volume has doubled. Then knead the dough again. Bake the yeast dough topped as a pizza 20-30 minutes at 200 degrees.

Waffles

Ingredients:

- ➤ 8 egg yolks, 8 tablespoons sunflower oil (or omega 3)
- ➤ 8 tablespoons protein powder, 4 tablespoons yogurt (or curd)
- ➤ 8 tablespoons water (or cream), 1 sachet of baking powder

Procedure: Bake the waffles in the waffle iron until golden brown. The wafers can be frozen arranged in layers (aluminum foil in between) and then toasted in the toaster (or oven). They can be sweetened with (please, no sugar), cottage cheese, yogurt, or even with cheese or sausage.

Almond Carrot Cake

Ingredients:

- ➤ 250 g carrots cut small, 4 eggs, stir the egg whites stiff
- ➤ 4 tsp liquid sweetener, 400 g ground almonds, A pinch of salt

Procedure: Mix all ingredients and finally fold in the eggs. Pour into the muffin-shaped and bake at approximately 175 degrees for about 40-45 minutes.

Nut Cake

Ingredients:

- ➤ 7 egg yolks, 200 g ground walnuts
- ➤ 1 teaspoon baking aroma of bitter almonds, 4 tablespoons liquid sweetener

Procedure: Separate the eggs. Stir the egg yolk with the bitter aroma very fluffy, then sweeten with 2 tsp sweetener. Stir the egg-white until stiff and sweeten with 2 tsp too. Fold half of the egg whites in the yolks and then add the nuts and the remaining snow. Stir carefully, otherwise the snow collapses. Now place the mixture in a greased ring tin and bake for about 50 minutes in the oven at about 165 degrees. Then leave it 15 minutes of cool-off before we can overthrow it.

The cake can be filled with whipped cream! 1/4 liter whipping cream, 2 teaspoons unsweetened cocoa powder, sweetener. Stir at will with cocoa cream until stiff and sweeten at last.

Cheesecake

Ingredients:

For the base:

> ➤ 80 g butter, 170 g ground almonds, 20 g wheat bran (or spelt bran)

> ➤ 80 g protein powder, 1 vanilla flavoring powder, 2 tablespoons liquid sweetener, 1 sachet baking powder

Procedure: Mix the dough well, it crumbles a bit. Put this mass (crumbs) into a greased springform pan and press down.

Ingredients:

For the topping:

> ➤ 4 eggs, 3 egg whites, 800 g quark

> ➤ flavor baking vanilla, 4 tablespoons liquid sweetener

> ➤ 1 packet jelly, no matter what flavor (no sugar)

Procedure: Stir the seven egg whites until stiff. Mix the egg yolks with the sweetener and the Jell-O powder. Then fold the egg whites in. Put the dough on the base dough. Cover with aluminum foil for the first 35 minutes, then take the foil away and bake until the end at 160 degrees about 70 minutes.

Then cut the oven off and cool about 20-30 minutes in the closed oven.

Amaretto Cookies

Ingredients:

- 100 g soft butter, 4 tablespoons liquid sweetener
- 2 egg yolks, 1 whole egg, 3 tablespoons amaretto liqueur
- A few drops of bitter almond flavor baking and vanilla flavor baking
- 80 g ground almonds, 50 g protein powder, 2 teaspoons baking powder

Procedure: Stir butter and liquid ingredients until creamy. Mix almonds, protein powder and baking powder and knead into dough. Put the dough in the fridge for half an hour, then form small balls and arrange them on a baking sheet covered with baking paper and flatten slightly. Bake in the preheated oven at 180 degrees for 15-20 minutes.

Bounty Cake

Ingredients:

- 200 g desiccated coconut, 4 tablespoons oil
- 6 heaping tablespoons cocoa, 4 eggs, 1 teaspoon baking powder
- 5 tsp sweetener, 6 large tablespoons cottage cheese

Procedure: First mix all dry ingredients, then add the wet ingredients and stir. Cook seven minutes in the microwave.

Marzipan Cake

Ingredients:

- 250 g melted butter, 4 egg yolks, 150 g ground almonds
- 3 heaped tablespoons protein powder, 1 baking aroma of bitter almonds, 4 tablespoons liquid sweetener, ½ sachet of baking powder

Procedure: Mix butter, eggs, sweetener, almonds and protein powder, and finally add the flavor. Stir it well. Pour into a cake pan and bake about 40 minutes at 180 degrees.

Tiramisu

Ingredients:

- ➢ 5 tablespoons ground coffee, 1 baking vanilla flavoring, 2 eggs
- ➢ 3 tablespoons Cognac, 170 g low fat curd cheese
- ➢ 80 g biscuits (recipe like seen above), 2 teaspoons cocoa

Procedure: Cook a very strong coffee and let it cool, separate eggs and stir egg whites until stiff. Leave to chill.

Put egg yolk, vanilla and brandy flavoring back into a mixing bowl and stir it in a hot water bath into a thick cream mix. Leave to chill. Then stir the egg whites with the cream until smooth. Stir the low fat curd cheese until creamy and stir in the egg-cream. Dip the biscuits briefly in cold coffee. Cover a baking-dish with half the biscuits and arrange half of the cream on it. Lay other cookies on it. Arrange the rest of the cream on it and sift the cocoa on it. Chill three hours in the fridge.

Philadelphia cake

Ingredients:

- ➢ 600 g cream cheese, Stir 250 ml cream until stiff
- ➢ 1 packet jelly (no sugar, no matter what flavor)
- ➢ Melt 200 g butter, 350 g ground almonds, 4 tablespoons sweetener

Procedure: Stir in the jelly in a little water and heat to dissolve. Mix it in the cream cheese and add 4 tablespoons of liquid sweetener. Then fold in the whipped cream.

For the base:

Ingredients:

- ➢ 200 g melted butter, 340 g ground almonds

Procedure: Stir ingredients crumbly and fill it on the bottom of a springform tin, press until smooth and chill.

Then put the jelly-type material on it. Chill about 4 to 5 hours in the fridge.

Spice cake

Ingredients:

- 250 g melted butter, 5 tablespoons liquid sweetener
- Stir 6 eggs until fluffy, 1 teaspoon ground coriander
- 2 tablespoons cocoa, 1 teaspoon cinnamon
- 1 teaspoon ground cloves, Or use gingerbread spice!
- 1 baking aroma of vanilla 100 protein powder
- 200 g ground almonds, 1 packet of baking powder

Procedure: Mix ingredients. Put the dough in a greased (and sprinkled with almonds) springform and bake at 160 degrees about 50 to 60 minutes. Melt a cube for the chocolate glaze and add 3 tablespoons cream, 1 teaspoon cocoa and 2 teaspoons liquid sweetener. Mix well and arrange it in two layers on the still warm cake.

Cherry gateau

Ingredients:

- Whip 4 egg whites until stiff, 4 egg yolks
- 100g ground almonds, 2 teaspoons liquid sweetener
- 2 tablespoons cocoa, 1 teaspoon baking powder

Procedure: Mix egg yolks with the sweetener and mix with the almonds, cocoa and baking powder in the whipped egg whites. Cover a spring form with baking paper and arrange the dough. Bake about 35 minutes at 180 degrees on the center rack. Put the cold base in a pie plate and place around a cake edge.

Ingredients:

- Whip 500 ml cream until stiff, 2 teaspoons liquid sweetener
- 1 baking aroma vanilla, 6 gelatine leaves (and some extra gelatine for the cherries)
- 1 jar of cherries, For the chocolate chips you need 75% strong chocolate

Procedure: Drain the cherries and set aside 16 cherries. Thicken the juice slightly with the gelatine. After cooling, stir in the cherries and a glass of cherry brandy. Arrange the cherry mixture on the cold base. Soak the gelatine can be crushed and melt in a cup in a water bath. Whip the cream, fold the sweetener, baking aroma of vanilla and gelatine into the cream and arrange it with the cherries on baked pastry case. Put the cake for 4-5 hours in the refrigerator. Before serving, re-move cake edge and decorate the edge with grated chocolate. Mark 16 pieces and put the cherries as decoration on it.

Chocolate Cream

Ingredients:

➢ 200 g cottage cheese, 1 teaspoon cocoa

➢ 4 tablespoons cream, 2 tablespoons liquid sweetener

Procedure: Mix the ingredients. 3 days nonperishable in the fridge.

Advocaat Torte

For the base:

Ingredients:

➢ Stir 4 egg whites until stiff, 4 egg yolks

➢ 150g ground almonds, 1 tablespoon egg white powder

➢ A few drops of vanilla flavoring, 2 teaspoons liquid sweetener

Procedure: Mix egg yolks with the sweetener and lift in the beaten egg whites with the ingredients. Pour into a baking tray and bake at 180 degrees about 30 minutes.

Covering:

Ingredients:

➢ 4 egg yolks, 2 teaspoons liquid sweetener

➢ 200 g eggnog, 7 sheets gelatin, 500 ml whipping cream stiff-stirred

Procedure: Whip egg yolks, 4 tablespoons sweetener and eggnog until creamy. Add remaining eggnog. Dissolve soaked gelatine in low heat, mix it with the egg yolk mixture and chill. Whip cream until stiff. Once the egg yolk mixture begins to thicken, fold in whipped cream and spread on the ground. Arrange a little eggnog on the solidified mass. The whole thing about 4-5 hours in the fridge.

Cream Cheese Cake

For the base:

Ingredients:

- ➢ 4 stiff egg whites, 4 egg yolks, 100g ground almonds
- ➢ 1 tablespoon egg white powder, A few drops of vanilla flavoring
- ➢ 2 teaspoons liquid sweetener

Procedure: Mix egg yolks with the sweetener and drag with the ingredients in the beaten egg whites. Pour into a baking tray and bake at 180 degrees (medium bar) about 30 minutes.

Covering:

Ingredients:

- ➢ 100 g melted butter, 3 teaspoons liquid sweetener
- ➢ 1 packet vanilla flavoring, 3 eggs, separated (egg whites until stiff)
- ➢ 500 g low-fat quark, 6 soaked gelatine leaves, 250 ml stiff cream

Procedure: Stir vanilla flavoring, a pinch of salt and butter with the sweetener and the egg yolks until fluffy. Add quark, baked vanilla and salt. Mix well. Press gelatine well and dissolve it in 2-3 tbsp hot water. Stir the still warm gelatine is in the quark mass. Fold in whipped cream and stiffly beaten egg snow.

Strawberry cream cake

For the base:

Ingredients:

- ➢ 4 stiff egg whites, 4 egg yolks, 100g ground almonds
- ➢ 1 tablespoon egg white powder, A few drops of vanilla flavoring
- ➢ 2 teaspoons liquid sweetener

Procedure: Mix egg yolks with the sweetener and drag with the ingredients in the beaten egg whites. Pour into a baking tray and bake at 180 degrees about 30 minutes.

Covering:

Ingredients:

➤ 500 g fresh strawberries, 500 ml whipping cream

➤ 2 tsp liquid sweetener, 1 baking aroma of vanilla

➤ 100 ml apple juice, 6 soaked white gelatine leaves

Procedure: Puree half the strawberries. Put remaining strawberries aside. Stir cream, vanilla flavor and sweetener until stiff. Dissolve gelatine. Gradually stir in apple juice and stir the mixture with the strawberry puree. When the mixture begins to thicken, fold in whipped cream. 4-5 hours in the fridge.

Russian chocolate cheesecake

(aka "Zupfkuchen")

For the base:

Ingredients:

➤ 90 g melted (and a bit cooled) butter, 200 g ground almonds

➤ 20 g wheat bran, 70 g protein powder

➤ 4 teaspoons liquid sweetener, A few drops of vanilla flavoring

Procedure: The dough is crumbly, never mind. Give half of it (perhaps with ground almonds and breadcrumbs) in a greased springform pan (18 cm diameter) and press it. In a larger (normal) springform pan, the cake won't be that pretty high.

For the topping:

Ingredients:

➤ 2 frothy eggs (4 min), 500 g stirred cottage cheese

➤ 1 packet white instant gelatin, 4 tablespoons liquid sweetener

Procedure: Stir the ingredients, arrange the compound on the base and smooth it. Then put small flat spots from the other half (I added 1 heaped teaspoon cocoa and a little cream) on the cheese surface. Bake at 180 degrees about 1 hour. Turn off oven. I left the cake 10 minutes in the closed oven.

Cinnamon poppy seed or almond cake

Ingredients:

- ➤ 250 ml cream cheese, 200 g ground poppy seeds or almonds
- ➤ 70 g melted butter, 4 tablespoons liquid sweetener
- ➤ 1 teaspoon cinnamon, 1 teaspoon baking soda
- ➤ 30 g protein powder (vanilla), 6 eggs, 1 bottle of vanilla flavoring

Procedure: Stir the eggs until very foamy and add the rest of the ingredients. Stir and out it into a greased cake pan. Bake at 160 degrees 40-50 minutes.

Woodruff cake

For the base:

Ingredients:

- ➤ 90 g melted butter, 100 g of protein powder
- ➤ 200g ground almonds (that may also be in accordance with hazel-nuts.)
- ➤ 1 packet baking powder, 3 tablespoons liquid sweetener

Procedure: This dough is very crumbly, arrange the crumbs into the greased baking dish (a full-size form) and at first make a small edge and press the dough afterwards.

For the topping:

Ingredients:

- ➤ 4 eggs (stirred fluffy), Stir 1 kg of skimmed cheese with the eggs
- ➤ 2 packs Jelly woodruff taste, without sugar, 6 tablespoons liquid sweetener

Procedure: Mix together and place on the base dough. Bake the cake in a preheated oven at 180 degrees for one hour, then leave it in the shut down and closed oven for 15 to 25 minutes. It won't collapse, and a small piece of cake does well enough.

Chocolate muffins without protein powder!

Ingredients:

- ➢ 100 g melted butter, 6 very creamy stirred eggs
- ➢ 1 packet vanilla flavor, 1 packet of baking powder
- ➢ 400 g ground hazelnuts, 100 g bran
- ➢ 80 g sliced almonds (or coarsely chopped), 2 tablespoons ground coffee
- ➢ 2 tablespoons cream or very strong coffee, brew about half a cup yourself. Don't add cream then
- ➢ 2 heaped teaspoon cocoa, 5-6 tablespoons liquid sweetener

Procedure: Stir eggs until frothy and mix in remaining ingredients. Bake at 165 degrees about 40-45 minutes. You could also make biscuits of this receipt!

Microwave cake for Advent

Ingredients:

- ➢ 1 egg, 1 teaspoon cocoa, 2 tablespoons oil
- ➢ 120 g quark, 20 g ground almonds, 20 g protein powder
- ➢ 2 tablespoons liquid sweetener, 1 packet of gingerbread spice
- ➢ 2 teaspoons baking powder, a few drops of vanilla flavoring

Procedure: Stir egg until frothy, mix in the other ingredients and put it for about 3 minutes at 600 watts in the microwave. Instead of ginger-bread spice you can take almond biscuit spice or another spice mix of ground cloves, cardamom and cinnamon.

Poppy-quark-cake

Ingredients:

- ➢ Stir 6 eggs until fluffy, 200 g poppy seeds, 250 g cream cheese
- ➢ 60 g melted butter, 5 tsp liquid sweetener, 1 vial of vanilla baking aroma
- ➢ 1 level teaspoon soda, 30 g protein powder

Procedure: Stir eggs until very frothy and stir in remaining ingredients. Bake for about 45-50 minutes at 160 degrees and let it chill.

Browny Cake

Ingredients:

- ➤ 6 egg yolks, 300 g quark, 40 g desiccated coconut
- ➤ 160 g ground almonds, 40 g bran, 6 heaped teaspoons cocoa
- ➤ 2 level tsp baking soda, 2 level tsp vitamin C powder
- ➤ 600g grated carrots, 1 packet baking rum flavoring
- ➤ 1 packet baking aroma vanilla, 5 tablespoons liquid sweetener
- ➤ 1 pinch salt, 1 teaspoon coffee powder, 4 tablespoons protein powder
- ➤ 6 tablespoons vinegar, 1 tablespoon flax seed, 3 tsp cinnamon
- ➤ pinch of cardamom, 100 ml cream, 100 ml of red wine

If the dough is too dry, add some more cream.

Procedure: Spread dough on parchment paper (smeared with butter and sprinkled with ground almonds) in a spring-form and bake at 160 degrees about 30 - 45 minutes. Cool at room temperature.

Cake stand with Mascarpone Cream

Ingredients:

- ➤ 3 separated eggs, Beat egg whites until stiff
- ➤ 120 g ground almonds, 1 teaspoon protein powder
- ➤ 2 tablespoons liquid sweetener, ½ packet vanilla flavoring
- ➤ 1 pinch of salt, 1 teaspoon baking powder

Procedure: Stir egg whites with a pinch of salt and sweetener until stiff. Mix the ground almonds and baking powder with the egg yolk. Then fold in egg whites. Put the dough in a greased flan mold (with ground almonds) and bake at 160 degrees 25-30 minutes. Stir 250 g mascarpone with egg yolks and 1 tablespoon liquid sweetener until smooth and spread on the base.

OR: Spread 250 g frosted berries on the base and 250 g cream cheese mixed with 100 ml whipping cream and 2 tablespoons liquid sweetener and spread it on the berries.

Walnut waffles

Ingredients:

- ➢ 6 eggs stirred fluffy, 60 g ground walnuts
- ➢ 6 tablespoons oil, 8 tablespoons protein powder (more or less)
- ➢ 1 packet of baking powder, 1 baking vanilla flavoring
- ➢ 5 tablespoons liquid sweetener

Procedure: The dough must be thick. Separate the eggs and beat egg whites until stiff. Mix egg yolks with the remaining ingredients and fold in the stiff egg whites. Bake until Yellow Gold.

Almond Pancakes

Ingredients:

- ➢ 3 frothy mixed eggs, 5 tablespoons of ground almonds
- ➢ 3 tablespoons cream (more or less), 3 teaspoons liquid sweetener
- ➢ 1 pinch of salt, 1 tablespoon egg white powder

Procedure: The dough should be slightly thick. Stir eggs until frothy and stir in remaining ingredients. Make small pancakes in a hot frying pan.

Semolina

Ingredients:

- ➢ 100 ml cream, 100 ml water, 5 tablespoons ground almonds
- ➢ A few drops of vanilla flavoring, 2 tablespoons liquid sweetener
- ➢ 1 tablespoon egg white powder

Procedure: Mix very fine with the immersion blender. Heat two minutes in the microwave for a warm cream of wheat.

Coconut macaroons

Ingredients:

> ➤ Stir 5 egg whites until stiff. Mix with, 1 teaspoon lemon powder and

> ➤ 5 tablespoons sweetener (powder), Fold under 200 g coconut flakes.

Procedure: Makes 8-9 large coconut macaroons on a plate! Bake about 45 minutes at 125 degrees in the oven, let cool then in the closed oven for 15-20 minutes.

Cookies without protein powder

Ingredients:

> ➤ 150 g butter, melted, 4 egg yolks, 50 g ground walnuts

> ➤ 50 g ground flaxseed, 50 g ground sesame

> ➤ 200 g ground almonds, 100 g ground hazelnuts, (everything ground in a coffee grinder)

> ➤ 1 sachet baking powder, 1 teaspoon cocoa

> ➤ 3 - 4 drops of peppermint oil (from the pharmacy)

Procedure: Roll small balls and flatten slightly. Bake at 180 degrees 20-25 minutes.

Advent Cookies

Ingredients:

> ➤ 6 egg yolks, 200 g butter, melted, 1 packet of baking powder

> ➤ 8 tsp liquid sweetener, Gingerbread spice (or coffee or cinnamon or?)

> ➤ 200 g ground almonds, 200 g of protein powder

Procedure: Stir the whole thing a few minutes. Form small balls and flatten. Then place on a baking paper on a tray. Bake 30 minutes at 180 degrees.

Micro-walnut cookies

Ingredients:

> ➢ 100 g ground walnuts, 1 baking vanilla flavoring

> ➢ 2 tablespoons butter, 2 tablespoons liquid sweetener

Procedure: Cook in microwave about 3 minutes. Topping: Sprinkle whipped cream (no sugar) and cinnamon.

Biscuit biscuits in microwave or oven

Ingredients:

> ➢ 4 fluffy stirred eggs, 40 g bruised flaxseed grain

> ➢ 60 g ground almonds, 1 tsp cinnamon, 3 tsp liquid sweetener

> ➢ 120g mascarpone, 1 tbsp protein powder

Procedure: Stir eggs until frothy and stir remaining ingredients into the batter. Swell the dough about 10 minutes. Cut parchment paper to fit in microwave dish. Put small heaps on it using a tablespoon. Be careful, the dough still smudges. Cook in the microwave at 900 watts for about 5 minutes. Or: In a springform pan (parchment paper) and bake at 180 degrees 25-30 minutes in the oven. The dough should still be very light brown. That can also be a pie crust!

Peanut Butter Cookies

Ingredients:

½ cup peanut butter with pieces (without sugar)

200 g mascarpone, 100 g chopped nuts

1 packet vanilla flavoring, 4 tablespoons liquid sweetener

1 tablespoon egg white powder, 1 teaspoon baking powder

Procedure: Place all ingredients in a bowl, mix well. Put biscuits with a teaspoon (don't forget baking paper!) on a baking sheet and bake 12-16 minutes.

Saint Nick's Cookies

Ingredients:

- ➤ 5 egg whites, 5 tablespoons liquid sweetener
- ➤ 250 g ground almonds, 50 g protein powder
- ➤ 1 teaspoon cinnamon, 1 heaped teaspoon cocoa, 1 pinch of cloves
- ➤ 1 dash lemon juice and orange juice (for the glaze)

Procedure: Beat egg whites until stiff, set about ¼ aside for later brushing. Gradually knead in the remaining ingredients. Roll out dough and cut into slices. Put the slices on the baking sheet (with paper, of course...). Make a spreadable glaze out of the egg white and the juice and brush the slices (cookies). Bake about 30 to 40 minutes at 180 degrees.

Almond heaps

Ingredients:

- ➤ 200 g chopped almonds, 5 egg whites
- ➤ 1 pinch of salt, 4 tablespoons liquid sweetener

Procedure: Stir protein with the sweetener until stiff and mix with the almonds. Give piles on a baking sheet (with paper). Bake 15-20 minutes at 165 degrees.

Vanilla crescents

Ingredients:

- ➤ 175 g ground almonds, 1 teaspoon baking powder
- ➤ 3 teaspoons liquid sweetener, 2 tablespoons protein powder (more or less), 1 egg, 2 tablespoons sour cream
- ➤ 120 g soft butter, 1 sachet vanilla flavoring

Procedure: Knead all ingredients into a dough and chill in the fridge about 2 hours. Form in portions to a role and place small crescents on the baking sheet (with parchment paper) at a distance of about 1 cm. Bake about 8-10 minutes in heated oven at 165 degrees. Let cool on the baking sheet and sprinkle a touch of sweetener.

Cinnamon stars

Ingredients:

- ➢ 5 egg whites, 5 tsp liquid sweetener
- ➢ 250 g ground almonds, 50 g protein powder
- ➢ 1 pinch salt, 2 tsp cinnamon, ½ packet rum flavoring

Procedure: Stir the egg whites until stiff and put aside about ¼ of it for brushing. Mix sweetener, almonds, protein powder and cinnamon in the egg white and make a dough. Roll out the dough and cut out stars. Place on a baking sheet (with paper). Make a spreadable glaze with the rest of the whipped egg whites, add a little rum and brush the surface of the star with it. Bake at 175 degrees for 20-30 minutes

Advent chocolates

Ingredients:

- ➢ 50 g "hard fat" cooking fat, 100 g butter, 2 tablespoons cocoa, 200 g cream
- ➢ 4 tablespoons coconut flakes, 4 teaspoons liquid sweetener

Procedure: Melt butter and "hard fat", add the rest and stir. Then fill in small paper forms (for chocolate) and chill (durable 3 days).

Shortbread

Ingredients:

- ➢ 30 g soft butter, 1 pinch of salt, juice and paring of 1/2 lemon
- ➢ 3 tablespoons liquid sweetener, 3 eggs, 200 g cottage cheese
- ➢ 3 tablespoons protein powder (more or less), 1 packet of baking soda

Procedure: Knead all ingredients to a dough. Fill the thickish batter into a pastry bag with a suitable nozzle and spray the little squiggles on a baking sheet covered with parchment paper. Bake at 175 degrees 9-12 minutes.

Gingerbread

Ingredients:

- ➢ 70 g melted butter, 3 eggs, 130g ground almonds
- ➢ 70 g egg whites, 2 tablespoons baking cocoa
- ➢ 1/3 tsp vanilla flavor, gingerbread spice
- ➢ 1 teaspoon baking soda, 3 tablespoons liquid sweetener

Procedure: Form a stiff dough and flat biscuits and bake at 180 degrees about 25 minutes.

Cinnamon rolls

Ingredients:

- ➢ 125 g melted butter, 3 egg yolks, 2 teaspoons sweetener
- ➢ 1 teaspoon cinnamon, 1 teaspoon cocoa
- ➢ 2 tablespoons protein powder, 200 g ground almonds
- ➢ ½ teaspoon baking powder, 1 pinch of salt, 30 ml milk
- ➢ ½ teaspoon cinnamon, 1 tablespoon egg white powder, ½ vanilla flavoring

Procedure: Mix all ingredients and place the dough in the foil about 2 hours in the refrigerator. Out of the whole shape dough into a roll and form 50 balls and place on a sheet lined with parchment paper and press on. Brush the cookies with the cast. Put back in the preheated oven at 170 degrees about 7 minutes. Durable in a can as long as "normal" biscuits.

Black and white cookies

Ingredients:

- ➢ 6 tablespoons protein powder (more or less)
- ➢ 6 tbsp ground almonds, 1 teaspoon baking powder
- ➢ 4 teaspoons liquid sweetener, ½ teaspoon baking rum flavoring
- ➢ 180 g soft butter, 1 vanilla flavoring

Procedure: Knead all the ingredients, then knead half of the dough with the 2 tablespoons cocoa and 2 tablespoons water. Roll out both doughs evenly thick, lay them on each other and press lightly. Roll up from one side and cut into slices. Put the cookies on the sheet (with parchment paper) and bake at 160 degrees about 12 minutes.

Berry-quark gratin

Ingredients:

- ➢ 3 eggs, ½ tbsp lemon, 150 g quark
- ➢ 300 g berries, 3 tsp liquid sweetener
- ➢ 2 tablespoons cream, 1 vanilla flavoring

Procedure: Separate the eggs for the quark mass. Stir yolks and sweetener until fluffy. Mix lemon juice, cottage cheese and cream. Stir egg whites until stiff, add vanilla and baking aroma and make a thick mass. Gently fold into the quark mass. Grease a baking dish, pour the quark mass and add the berries. Bake 25 minutes - at 175 degrees about 20 minutes.

Rocket-walnut-quark

Ingredients:

- ➢ 500 g quark, 3 tablespoons cream
- ➢ 50 g rocket, 15 walnut halves
- ➢ salt and pepper, 1 tsp liquid sweetener

Procedure: Stir the cheese and the cream until creamy, season with salt, pepper and sweetener. Wash arugula and cut it into thin strips, crumble the walnuts, mix them and chill a few hours.

Jam

Ingredients:

- ➢ 600 g of fruit (berries, pears, apples)
- ➢ 1 packet gelatine (immediately soluble)
- ➢ 6 tablespoons liquid sweetener

Procedure: Puree the fruit, put it in a saucepan, stir it into the gelatine and add sweetener. Boil stirring 2 to 3 minutes, then pour into jars and cool. 2 - 3 hours in the fridge, and the mass is firm.

Pudding

Ingredients:

- ➢ 200 ml soy milk, 200 ml water
- ➢ 60 g coconut flakes, ½ teaspoon cinnamon
- ➢ 2 tablespoons liquid sweetener, 2 tablespoons baking powder
- ➢ 1 egg white, vanilla flavoring, Gelatine for ½ liters of fluid

Procedure: Mix well and heat in a saucepan. Add gelatine, fill in a small bowl and put in the refrigerator for about 4-5 hours.

Amaretto ice cream

Ingredients:

- ➢ 400 ml cream, 200 g sour cream,
- ➢ 50 g ground almonds, 1 jigger Amaretto
- ➢ 3 tablespoons baking powder, 1 egg white vanilla flavoring

> ½ teaspoon baking aroma of bitter almonds

> 5 teaspoons liquid sweetener

Procedure: Roast ground almonds until they are lightly browned and stir into the mixture. Mix all ingredients with a whisk and put it into the ice machine, or freeze it about 5 - 6 hours.

Ice Sorbet

Ingredients:

> 350 g frozen berries, 1 cup sour cream

> ½ cup yogurt, 2 tablespoons liquid sweetener

Procedure: Puree frozen fruit in the blender. Mix all ingredients. You can freeze it a few days but not longer than one week. Take out of the fridge ca. ½ hour before serving

Strawberry ice cream

Ingredients:

> 500 g strawberries, Juice of one lemon

> 4 tablespoons liquid sweetener

> 500 g cream cheese

Procedure: Puree strawberries, mix with cream cheese. Freeze in a plastic box about 5 hours. Take out 15 minutes before consumption.

Buttermilk ice

Ingredients:

> 500 ml butter milk, 4 tablespoons liquid sweetener

> 250 ml whipped cream

> Grated lemon and orange peel

Procedure: Mix buttermilk, cream, sweetener and finely grated rind of half a lemon and a half of orange and freeze well. Then put it in the ice machine and wait until the mixture is creamy. Or freeze for 4 - 5 hours.

Mocha Ice

Ingredients:

- ➢ 250 g quark, 2 egg yolks, 4 tablespoons liquid sweetener
- ➢ Dissolve 3 teaspoons instant coffee, 125 g cream
- ➢ 1 egg white, ½ vanilla flavoring Back

Procedure: Whip cream until stiff, beat egg whites until stiff and mix them together. Now fill in the quark mass and the cream mass in layers.

Chocolate ice cream

Ingredients:

- ➢ 6 eggs, 3 teaspoons cocoa powder
- ➢ 250 ml cream, 4 tablespoons liquid sweetener
- ➢ 3 dashes of rum flavoring

Procedure: Separate eggs and beat egg whites until stiff, beat cream until stiff. Whisk egg yolks, cocoa, sweetener, baking rum flavoring, carefully fold a third of stiff egg whites, mix and fold in the remaining egg whites and then the cream. Pour into 7 small freezing boxes and freeze in the refrigerator for about 4 hours.

Raffaelos

Ingredients:

- ➢ 125 g coconut oil, 125 g butter
- ➢ 250 g coconut flakes, 1 bottle essence of bitter almonds
- ➢ 4 tablespoons liquid sweetener, 50 ml cream

Procedure: Melt coconut oil and butter. Stir in 150 g coconut flakes, essence of bitter almonds, cream and sweetener. Let cool. When the mixture is almost set, make balls and roll in remaining coconut flakes. Store in a refrigerator.

Chocolates

Ingredients:

> 150 g chocolate, high cocoa content

> 40 g whole nuts, 200g mascarpone cheese

> 4 tablespoons liquid sweetener

> 30 g Cocoa, 10 ml rum, 4 drops vanilla essence

Procedure: Melt chocolate and apply some at the edge of about 30 chocolates capsules. Turn them around to expire and allow to harden completely. Mix mascarpone, cocoa, rum, sweetener and vanilla essence. Fill each capsule with a nut and with mascarpone cream. In the refrigerator to harden. Then remove the cartridge and paper. Keep in the refrigerator.

Lemon Mousse

Ingredients:

> 2 eggs stirred frothy, 200 ml cream

> 2 lemons, 3 sheets gelatine

> 4 tablespoons liquid sweetener

Procedure: Soak gelatine in cold water, stir egg yolks and sweetener until fluffy. Grate ½ lemon and add the juice. Remove gelatine and press out the water. Mix with 3 tablespoons hot water until it is completely liquid. Add while stirring to the egg mixture and let chill. Stir occasionally. After about half an hour to (cream is still liquid), beat the protein and then the cream very stiff and carefully fold into the cream. 5 hours in the fridge

Homemade chocolate

Ingredients:

- ➤ 200 g coconut oil, 50 g butter
- ➤ 2 tablespoons cocoa powder
- ➤ 30 g ground hazelnuts, ½ Almond flavoring
- ➤ 4 tablespoons liquid sweetener

Procedure: Pour into muffin- or chocolate cups and put them 5 hours in the refrigerator.

Jelly

Brew ½ liter of tea using 6 tea bags (any flavor)

10-13 minutes brewing-time

5 tsp liquid sweetener

Dissolve 1 packet powdered gelatine in it and freeze it.

Nibbler Replacement

Almonds, peanuts, chocolate 85% cocoa

Cheese Chips

Cut parchment paper to the size of dinner plates. Cut the cheese slices into pieces and arrange them on the baking paper. Place not too tight since the cheese will run. Then bake for 4-5 minutes at 800 watts or 900 watts in the microwave.

It works as well in the oven!

Bacon chips

1 packet Bacon Ham

Cut a long strip into 5 pieces and place the pieces on paper towels.

Leave in the microwave until the bacon crackles no longer, 3 - 4 minutes at 900 watts. Or fry the whole crispy strips in a lot of oil in the pan! Pan must be very hot, pour the oil into it until hot and carefully put the ham strips in.

Pina Colada Cream

Ingredients:

> ➤ 500 g cottage cheese, 6 tablespoons shredded coconut

> ➤ 2 tsp pineapple syrup (KH-free), a few drops of rum flavoring

Procedure: Mix well and put it in the refrigerator.

Custard apple with nuts

Ingredients:

> ➤ 2 apples, 1 tbsp lemon juice

> ➤ 3 tablespoons chopped hazelnuts

> ➤ 1 tablespoon sliced almonds

> ➤ 1 tablespoon butter, 2 tsp cinnamon

> ➤ A few drops of vanilla flavoring

> ➤ 300 g of natural yogurt, 4 tablespoons liquid sweetener

Procedure: Peel the apples, quarter and remove the seeds. Cut the quarters crosswise into thin flakes and immediately sprinkle with lemon juice. Save1 teaspoon hazelnuts for garnish! Roast the nuts in a nonstick pan without fat until golden brown and put them aside. Melt the butter in a pan and fry the apples in it while stirring. Dust with cinnamon. Fold the custard apples in the yogurt and sweeten with sweetener. Sprinkle with hazelnuts.

Coconut sweets

Ingredients:

- ➤ 75 g melted butter, 15 g coconut oil
- ➤ 175 g condensed milk, 200 g desiccated coconut
- ➤ 3 teaspoons liquid sweetener

Procedure: Melt the fat, add the coconut flakes and mix. Add the condensed milk and the sweetener and cook another 10 minutes, stirring. Remove the pan from the heat and let the coconut mixture cool slightly. Sculpt the cooled mixture in long blocks and cut them into equal-sized rectangles. About 3 hours to cool down.

Mascarpone cream with pineapple and nuts

Ingredients:

- ➤ 200 g mascarpone cheese, 1 tbsp protein powder
- ➤ 100 ml cream (and maybe some water)
- ➤ 60 g coconut flakes, a dash of lemon juice, 100 g coarsely chopped nuts
- ➤ 1 slice of pineapple (from a no sugar can)

Procedure: Mix the mascarpone with the liquids, then stir in the remaining ingredients.

Peppermint Chocolate

Ingredients:

- ➤ 50 g chocolate (85% cocoa), 50 g "hard fat" cooking fat
- ➤ 1 vanilla flavoring, 50 ml cream
- ➤ 5 drops peppermint oil (from the pharmacy)
- ➤ 3 tablespoons liquid sweetener

Procedure: Melt the chocolate and "hard fat" and stir in the other ingredients. Then pour the whole thing into a chocolate mold and place in the fridge for 4 hours.

Grapefruit bowls with nuts

Ingredients:

- ➤ 1 large pink grapefruit, 150 g cottage cheese
- ➤ 2 tablespoons chopped nuts, 2 tablespoons liquid sweetener
- ➤ 150 g quartered sourish apples

Procedure: Halve the grapefruit. Detach the fruit fillets between the separating skins (creating two bowls). Collect the juice. Mix the cheese with the grapefruit juice, nuts and sweetener. Cut the apple-quarters crosswise into small pieces and fold into the curd. Fill the apple quark in the grapefruit bowls and arrange the grapefruit fillets on top of them.

Savoury Spreads

Ingredients:

- ➤ 100 g sour cream, 100 ml cream, 100 g yogurt
- ➤ 100 g quark, Garlic, pepper, salt, herbs

Procedure: Mix everything well with a whisk. Add garlic, pepper, salt and herbs. Stir the whole thing with a whisk until creamy. The creamy mass stays fresh 3 days in refrigerator.

Sausage salad

Ingredients:

- ➤ 750 g sausages (any variety), cut into small pieces
- ➤ 6 eggs (boiled) in small pieces, 4 tomatoes cut into small pieces
- ➤ 8 large pickles (pickles sweetened with artificial sweetener)
- ➤ 100 g mayonnaise, 1 large onion cut small
- ➤ 2 small red pepper cut small, salt, vinegar, oil, dried parsley

Procedure: Mix well and chill.

Fried cauliflower (or other vegetables)

Ingredients:

- ➢ Cook 1 cauliflower (Place in a baking dish)
- ➢ 500 g ground beef, 2 peppers, 1 onion, 1 carrot
- ➢ Curry, pepper, salt, pepper, oregano
- ➢ 1 can tomatoes, 250 ml cream

Procedure: Fry the meat with the ingredients. Drizzle over the cauliflower and bake with cheese (whatever) in the oven at 200 degrees for 45 minutes.

Stuffed tomatoes with tuna

Ingredients:

- ➢ Hollow out 4 large tomatoes
- ➢ Tuna from the can

Procedure: Fill the tomatoes with the tuna. Serve with salad and grained bread.

Stuffed peppers

Ingredients:

- ➢ 4 peppers, 500 g ground beef
- ➢ 1 egg, Curry, salt, pepper, paprika
- ➢ Chop 1 onion, Mince 2 cloves garlic
- ➢ Perhaps some fresh herbs!

Procedure: Carefully cut the pepper in the lid. Wash and remove seeds inside. Mix the raw meat in a bowl with the egg, the spice, the onion and the garlic. Fill the peppers with it and fry in a pan, then cover it and cook gently about 40 minutes.

Or put the peppers in a baking dish, drizzle cheese on them and bake about 45 - 50 minutes.

False potato pancakes

Ingredients:

> ➤ 1 kohlrabi, 1 carrot, 1 onion, 1 clove garlic

> ➤ 1 egg, spices (pepper, salt, curry, paprika)

> ➤ 1 tablespoon sesame seeds, 1 tablespoon protein powder

Procedure: Chop everything small in the food processor and fold the egg, the sesame seeds and spices in a bowl into the mixture. Bake kohlrabi pancakes in the pan.

Moussaka without potatoes

Ingredients:

> ➤ 500 g aubergines, Olive oil (or other oil), 500 g minced meat

> ➤ 2 Onions, cut into rings, 1 clove garlic chopped

> ➤ 1 tablespoon tomato paste, 300 g canned pizza tomatoes

> ➤ Salt, pepper, curry powder, 250 ml cream, 2 eggs

> ➤ 100g grated parmesan cheese, 100 g other grated cheese

Procedure: Cut eggplant slices, spread on a board, sprinkle with salt and let draw water for 30 minutes. Then dab with a paper towel. Roast ground beef golden brown in olive oil, add spices, onion rings and garlic. When the onions are translucent, add tomato paste and diced tomatoes. Heat covered 15 minutes on low heat. Take minced meat mixture from the pan and fry the eggplant in olive oil until golden brown. Brush a dish with butter and spread half the meat filling on the dish ground. Arrange the eggplant slices on top and put the second half of the filling on it. Mix cream, eggs and spices with a whisk and add the grated cheese. Drizzle this mixture over the moussaka. Bake at 180 degrees in the oven for about 40-45 minutes.

Mushroom pan

Ingredients:

200 g mushrooms (chanterelles or oyster mushrooms)

150 g cooked ham cubes, 4 slices of cheese

Salt, pepper, cayenne pepper, curry, paprika

1 chopped onion, 1 chopped clove garlic

Procedure: Fry mushrooms and sausage cubes in a little hot oil, salt and pepper. After about 2 minutes, add the cheese on top. Turn the hot plate a bit down and melt the cheese.

Asparagus ham rolls

Ingredients:

- ➤ 8 slices ham, 8 slices of cheese, 4 eggs
- ➤ 100 ml cream, 200 g grated cheese, 1-2 glasses of asparagus
- ➤ salt, pepper, curry, paprika, garlic powder

Procedure: Place cheese slices and 2-3 asparagus rolls on the ham slices, wrap and place in a baking dish. Stir the eggs, add a little cream, season and pour it over the rolls. Sprinkle the grated cheese at 180 degrees and heat the whole thing about 20-25 minutes in the oven.

Mincemeat muffins

Ingredients:

- ➤ 1 diced onion, 1 finely chopped clove garlic
- ➤ 1 red bell pepper cut into cubes, 150 g mushrooms
- ➤ 1 chopped bunch of parsley, 2 eggs, 400 g minced
- ➤ 1 pinch chili powder, 1 teaspoon mustard
- ➤ Salt and pepper, 1 teaspoon curry powder
- ➤ 1 dash lemon juice, 100 g cheese, Grease muffin pans well with oil!

Procedure: Mix the minced meat with all ingredients (except cheese) and pour into the muffin pans. Sprinkle with cheese and bake at 200 degrees about 40 minutes.

Minced meat pan with radishes

Ingredients:

- ➤ 500 g minced meat, 3 sliced onions, 2 chopped cloves garlic
- ➤ 1 quartered bunch radishes, 1 eggplant cut into cubes
- ➤ salt, pepper, curry, paprika, 1 tablespoon olive oil

Procedure: Fry all ingredients together in olive oil at low temperature (The radishes taste like potatoes).

Turkey roulade

Ingredients:

- ➤ 5 slices turkey cutlets, 5 slices of Leerdamer cheese
- ➤ 5 slices cooked ham, 1 can of tomatoes, 250g brunch
- ➤ 1 can of pizza tomatoes, 125 ml cream, 100 g grated cheese
- ➤ 1 chopped onion, 1 chopped clove garlic, Pepper, salt, curry, paprika

Procedure: Season the turkey steak. Put on every slice a slice of cheese and a slice of ham. Roll meat into a roulade and fry gently in very little oil. Arrange the meat in a baking dish. Mix tomatoes, onions and garlic with the brunch and the cream and pour it over the meat. Sprinkle with cheese. Cover the cutlets with aluminum foil for about 20 minutes. Heat at 175 degrees for about 40-45 minutes in the oven.

Salmon fillet with shrimp

Ingredients:

- ➤ 400 g frozen prawns, 400 g of frozen salmon fillets
- ➤ A few drops of lemon juice, Spices of your choice
- ➤ 250 ml cream, 60 g cream cheese, 80 g courgettes
- ➤ 200 g fresh tomatoes cut into thick slices
- ➤ 200g grated cheese, 5-6 garlic cloves

> ➤ 2 onions (cut into rings)

> ➤ 1 soup cube

Procedure: Let shrimps and salmon thaw. Season with lemon juice. Fry the salmon crispy, remove and place in a baking dish. Add prawns to the pan and fry. Once they absorb water, add the garlic, onion rings, cream, spices and bouillon cube, let it boil down slightly for about 10 minutes. Stir the cream cheese with a little water (or cream), and pour it into the mold. Now fry the zucchini a little in the pan and add it to the fish. Then drizzle the grated cheese over it. Finally, decorate with thick tomato slices. Scallop at 200 degrees for about 25-30 minutes.

Turkey burger

Ingredients:

> ➤ 200 g ground turkey, 1 cup of drained, frozen spinach

> ➤ Salt, pepper, a little nutmeg, curry, 1 egg

Procedure: Shape all ingredients into a burger and fry on both sides.

Pumpkin Curry Soup

Ingredients:

> ➤ 1 pumpkin, 2 soup cubes, 2 carrots cut small, 2 onions

> ➤ 1 clove garlic, 1 can coconut milk

> ➤ 1 shot orange juice, Spices, lots of curry!, 200 g sour cream

Procedure: Hollow the pumpkin out, put pumpkin meat aside. Boil pumpkin meat, onions, garlic and carrots with vegetable broth, spices and a splash of orange juice and cook it about 20 minutes. Then add coconut milk. Puree and season to taste with the spices. Add on top of each soup bowl a spoon of sour cream.

Spinach and cheese omelet

Ingredients:

> ➤ 1 onion, finely diced, 4 eggs

> ➤ Stew 1 clove garlic, finely chopped in 2 tablespoons olive oil in the pan

> ➤ 4 tablespoons thawed spinach, Parsley, salt, pepper, pinch of nutmeg

> ➤ 4 tablespoons mineral water, 100 g grated cheese

Procedure: Mix everything together and bake two pancakes. Put the pancakes on a baking sheet and sprinkle with cheese and bake for about 15 minutes in the oven at 200 degrees.

Cold chicken salad with pineapple

Ingredients:

> ➤ 500 g chicken cut into strips

> ➤ 3 slices of pineapple (or canned without sugar)

> ➤ 200 g mushrooms, 6 hard boiled eggs, 4 tablespoons sour cream

> ➤ 4 tablespoons mayonnaise, Chili seasoning, curry, salt, pepper

Procedure: Sear chicken with the spices and cook. Mix with the mayonnaise and other ingredients in a bowl.

Goat cheese with arugula

Ingredients:

> ➤ 300 g feta cheese, 100 g bacon (thin slices)

> ➤ ca. 200 g rocket parmesan cheese

> ➤ 3 tablespoons balsamic vinegar

> ➤ 3 tablespoons Olive oil

Procedure: Wash arugula and arrange it with balsamic vinegar and olive oil and spread on the plates. Sprinkle the parmesan cheese with a coarse cheese grater over it. Cut the sheep's cheese into cubes and wrap with bacon. Fry briefly in hot oil and turn until the bacon is browned on both sides. Garnish arugula salad with the cheese cubes.

Tuna Salad

Ingredients:

> ➤ 1 can of tuna, some olives, a few capers

> ➤ 1 onion, small cubed, 2 tablespoons olive oil

> ➤ a few drops of lemon juice, salt, pepper, curry, a little chili powder

Procedure: Drain the tuna. Cut olives into slices, fold onions, capers, lemon juice, olive oil, spices and into the tuna. Serve with lettuce.

Broccoli Salad

Ingredients:

> ➤ 500 g broccoli, shortly boiled, 1 cup sour cream

> ➤ 1 cup of cream, Pepper, salt, parsley, 1 dash lemon juice

> ➤ 1 red pepper, 200 g cooked ham (or else other sort of meat)

Procedure: Mix gently the cooled broccoli with sour cream, cream and spices. Dice the pepper and sauté lightly in butter. Cool and stir in the sour cream and pour over the broccoli mass. Cut the ham into cubes and add. Stir well once and chill a few hours in the fridge.

Cauliflower Salad

Ingredients:

> ➤ 1 small cauliflower (stew florets until al dente)

> ➤ 1 small cucumber, 2 red peppers, 1 onion,

> ➤ 1 clove of garlic, chopped, 3 slices cooked ham

> ➤ herbs, salt, pepper, vinegar, oil

Procedure: Cut peppers and ham into strips, add the remaining ingredients and mix well with the dressing.

Moroccan Coleslaw

Ingredients:

- ➤ 1 small white cabbage, 4 onions
- ➤ 1 clove garlic, 2 tablespoons oil, 2 tablespoons vinegar
- ➤ ½ tsp liquid sweetener, 3 tablespoons sesame seeds
- ➤ salt, pepper, 1 teaspoon mustard

Procedure: Cut all ingredients into small cubes. Mix the cabbage, the spices, the onions and the garlic with oil and vinegar and chill. Just before serving, add sesame seeds and mix salad gently again.

Cabbage salad with eggs

Ingredients:

- ➤ 350 g (or one can) sauerkraut, 1 cucumber
- ➤ 2 tomatoes, 1 onion, 1 clove garlic, 2 tablespoons vinegar
- ➤ 4 tablespoons oil, Salt, pepper, 1 teaspoon mustard
- ➤ 1 teaspoon liquid sweetener, 6 hard boiled eggs 1 bunch parsley

Procedure: Tear apart the sauerkraut and chop it. Peel the cucumber and cut it into small cubes. Scald the tomatoes briefly in hot water, remove the skin and dice. Cut the onions and garlic into thin rings. Mix a marinade from the vinegar and oil and season well with salt, pepper, mustard and sweetener. Mix the cabbage, cucumbers, tomatoes, put it in a salad bowl and fold in the marinade. Then peel and cube the eggs. Chop the herbs finely and mix with the eggs. Arrange the colorful sauerkraut salad and scatter the herbs-and-egg mixture on it.

White Bean Salad

Ingredients:

- ➢ 1 large onion, 3 cloves garlic, 250g cherry tomatoes
- ➢ 3 tablespoons olive oil, 2 tablespoons white wine
- ➢ 1 can white beans (400 g), 1 sprig rosemary
- ➢ 2 stalks thyme, 2 stalks of parsley salt, pepper, ½ tsp curry

Procedure: Cube onions and garlic finely. Wash tomatoes. Heat the olive oil in a shallow saucepan, sauté onions and garlic in it over medium heat while stirring. Add the whole tomatoes and cook for 5 minutes. Rinse the beans cold, add them and cook about 4 minutes. Chop the herbs finely, add salt and pepper to the beans. Before serving, drizzle with olive oil.

Minced meat with yogurt

Ingredients:

- ➢ 500 g minced meat, 250 g natural yoghurt, 2 tomatoes
- ➢ 3 gherkins, 1 onion, 1 apple - cut everything small.
- ➢ 1 tablespoon tomato paste, Salt, pepper

Procedure: Mix all in a bowl and put it in the pan. Braise it, always stirring. Serve with green beans or other vegetables.

Cucumber topped

Ingredients:

- ➢ 3 cucumbers, 500 g minced meat, 2 onions, 2 garlic cloves
- ➢ 200 g grated Gouda cheese (or other cheese), Pepper, salt, curry, paprika, some chili

Procedure: Halve the cucumbers and hollow them out. Cube the onion, the garlic and the inside of the cucumber and add to the minced meat. Season and mix. Fill the cucumber with the mixture and sprinkle with cheese. Place in a baking dish, add a little cream and bake for about 35 minutes in the oven at 200 degrees.

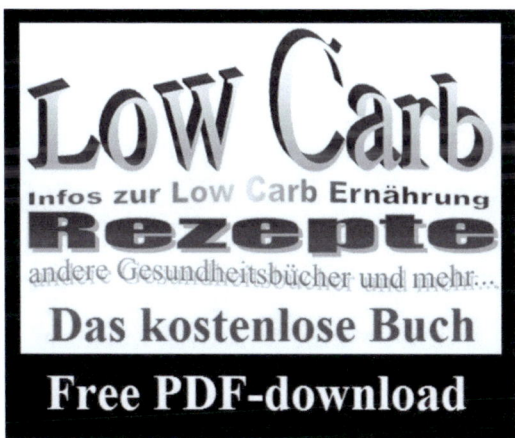

Lots of helpful information you can find inside this free pdf-book, use the following link.

http://www.jutta-schuetz-autorin.de/

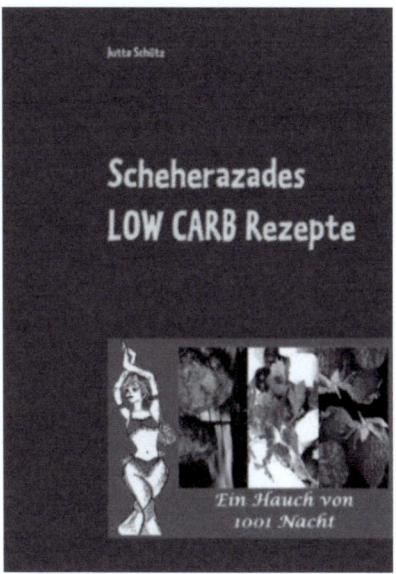

Scheherazades Low Carb Rezepte - 40 Orientalische Rezepte
ISBN-13: 978-3735737519
Books on Demand

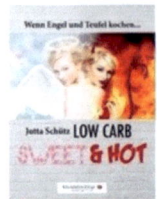

ISBN-13: 978-3981616576
A.S.Rosengarten-Verlag

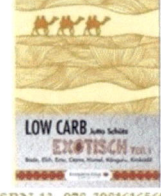

ISBN-13: 978-3981616569
A.S.Rosengarten-Verlag

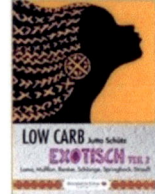

ISBN-13: 978-3981616569
A.S.Rosengarten-Verlag

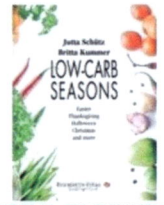

ISBN-13: 978-3981616514
A.S.Rosengarten-Verlag

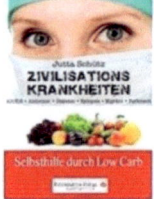

ISBN-13: 978-3981616521
A.S.Rosengarten-Verlag

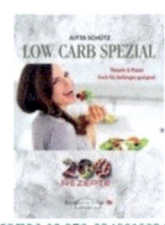

ISBN-13:978-3945015094
A.S.Rosengarten-Verlag

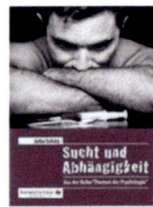

ISBN-13: 978-3945015056
A.S.Rosengarten-Verlag

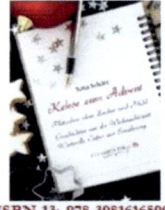

ISBN-13: 978-3981616590
A.S.Rosengarten-Verlag

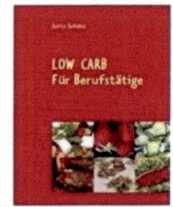

ISBN-13: 978-3732243280
Books on Demand

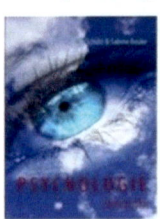

ISBN-13: 978-3732234929
Books on Demand

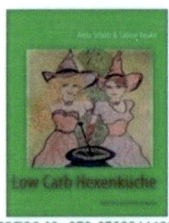

ISBN-13: 978-3732244621
Books on Demand

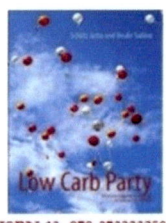

ISBN-13: 978-3732232505
Books on Demand

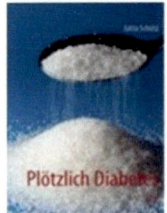

ISBN-13: 978-3732247721
Books on Demand

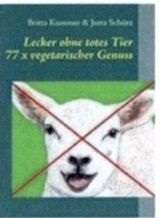

ISBN-13: 978-3842375406
Books on Demand

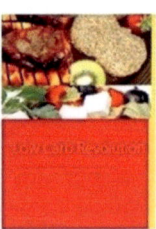

ISBN-13: 978-3844809084
Books on Demand